THE
AUTISM FITNESS HANDBOOK

Body Image • Motor Coordination • Posture
• Muscular Fitness • Cardiovascular Fitness

David S. Geslak, B.S., CSCS

The Autism Fitness Handbook
© 2011 David S. Geslak. All rights reserved.

ISBN: 978-0-615-47057-3

Exercise Connection Corporation
65 East Harris Avenue, Suite A2
La Grange, IL 60525

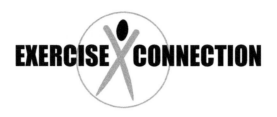

EXERCISE CONNECTION

THANK YOU . . .

....Mom and Dad for giving me the opportunities to help these children, families and organizations. Without your support I could not have done this. You are my heroes.

I love you.

...My family and friends: Danny, Tony, V, Deane, Lou, McCord, each of you have been there for me through many challenging times. Without each of you I would not have been able to stay focused and continue to help these children and families.

...My teachers and coaches: Mr. Papierski, Coach Doyle and the many teachers who have instilled the value of leadership, integrity and respect, because of which I have wanted to educate others and am sure glad I did.

....God, the power of prayer is amazing.

See the children for their capabilities, not their disabilities.
– David S. Geslak

Do you remember your grade school math teacher giving a test and saying, "First person to finish gets the best grade?" To some extent, this has been the philosophy behind physical education for the past 20 years. Since the 1980s, the way our children have been assessed in physical education (i.e., The President's Challenge) has not changed. The President's Challenge physical fitness test recognizes students for their level of fitness in sit-ups, the shuttle run, an endurance run/walk (the mile), pull-ups, push-ups, and the sit and reach. With these exercises, our children are being assessed on *quantity* of exercise (e.g., how many push-ups they do, how fast they run), not *quality* (e.g., proper form and body mechanics). When we work with the developing human body, this antiquated method of physical education does not support a child's physical needs. More importantly, this type of physical education does not meet the needs of a child with autism or any special needs. Each child should be considered unique, differing in size, shape, and ability. What can be considered notable progress for one child may not represent significant achievement for another. If we teach excesses and numbers, we are simply coaching, but not educating children about the human body or giving them a reason to enjoy physical activity.

For the past 20 years, we have seen changes detrimental to our children's physical development. Children as young as five-year-olds are being diagnosed with Type 2 diabetes, postural imbalances, obesity, heart disease, and, more recently, autism spectrum disorders. The physical needs of our children are changing. Most school administrators, parents, and students are aware of these changing needs, but there has been no change in how they are addressed. As Ed Arranga, founder of Autism One, once told me, "Raising awareness raises questions . . . increasing education provides answers."

The book and the Exercise Connection Program is focused on improving the health of children with autism as well as educating families and professionals about their role in making physical activity a part of their child's life. This book provides tips and tools necessary to implement an exercise program at home, in school or within any organization.

Each exercise will be described with an objective, how to, how many, coaching tips and a "bright idea" or interesting fact about the exercises. Each category is described below

Goal: The goal will describe the exercise's purpose and what you want to accomplish. This accomplishment/goal may take days, weeks, months or years depending on the ability of the child.

How To: This will give you a step-by-step approach to starting and ending the exercise.

How Many: This section will describe how many repetitions and sets should be done for each exercise. This is only a guideline. You will have to adapt to the ability of the child. A good reminder wil be: less is more.

Coaching Tips: This section will give you visual, verbal, sensory or tactile support tips that can help you to teach the exercise.

 The light bulb or "bright idea" will give alternatives to the exercise or educate you on why it is important to do.

Throughout the book, I will describe children with autism as children, youth, or students. Please recognize each of the descriptions as that of both a child and an adult. A majority of the exercises, activities, and protocols in the book have been used on children and adults. It is not as common for adults with autism to participate in exercise classes, so physically assess and begin their program as you would for a child. More challenging exercises can always be implemented as you move through their program. The structure of the class or individual session is a primary element to focus on, whether in an individual or group setting. Structure helps children and adults with autism understand your expectations and the challenges you set for them.

I'm often asked, "Is this program only for children with autism?" The answer is no. I have used the station setup for children of all abilities. The exercises can be used to help improve the cognitive and physical development of all children and adults.

The Exercise Connection Program has shown success with hundreds of children between the ages of 5 and 21, in small (2–5) and large groups (10–14) and in one-on-one sessions. The program has been implemented in both school settings and private training settings.

I reference group protocols in the book. These group protocols have been used during 45-minute sessions with up to 10 children in a class.

While this book is designed to provide you, your family and organization with a successful start, it is only a map. Each child and adult with autism is unique. What works one day, may not work the next day. A child may not like sports or a certain activity. Don't force the child to participate. Move on to one of their strengths, keep them engaged, and use your creativity as a mom, dad, big brother/sister, therapist or educator to make all activities a part of their program.

If your organization provides paraprofessionals for the children, make sure they read this manual. Not only is it important to have the parents' support and understanding of their child's exercise program, but anyone involved with these children must also understand the importance of physical activity.

Tips for Parents, Guardians, Caregivers, Schools, and Community Centers

1.   Be a leader

Most of you reading this are already leaders for children with autism, either as a parent or as an educator; however, are you a leader in their physical activity? I want parents to have another means of engaging with their child with autism. One day you may go into your basement for a quick workout, as your child with autism watches you leave – and one day your child with autism may *follow* you. You need to be the leaders in health and fitness. If your children see you participating, they may be more inclined to do so.

2.   Use your voice

At your children's schools, your voice needs to be heard on the issue of physical education. Explain the importance of physical activity to your parent/teacher organization and find out why the school administration does not make fitness programs a priority. During my talks with physical education teachers, they recognize the importance of such programs. Employ a team approach when advocating physical education, and make sure it is a part of your child's education.

3.   Assessments are positive

Many parents do not want to have their child's height and weight measured. They fear the child will be teased. Many schools honor the parents' wishes because the parents' voices are so strong. Physical assessments are not only about height and weight, but also about understanding the function and capabilities of your child's body. You should be educated on your child's health, and they should be too. Without an assessment and initial understanding of the child's body, how can you measure improvement and educate them about it?

4.   Music is great

Music is a huge motivator for a child with autism. If it works, use it, even if it is the same song for an hour. I cannot tell you how many times I have heard the song "Spoonful of Sugar" from the *Mary Poppins* soundtrack while working with one of my students. Each time I hear it, my smile gets bigger. Music is a huge motivator for many people when they go to the gym. Just look around at all the folks wearing iPods next time you are there.

5.   Family is strong

A chain is only as strong as its weakest link. At home, the family must work together to improve the health of the child in need. Dads, Moms, brothers, and sisters, physical activity gives you a means to connect with your child or sibling with autism. And remember, your actions are being watched – not just fitness activities, but everything including the food you put on the table. Your child with autism is observing every move you make.

There is no better time than now to start educating our children about physical activity. Our children should not be forced into physical activity, nor should it be used as a form of punishment (e.g., "go run a lap"). Physical activity is a way for our children to let their bodies be free, rid themselves of toxins, and improve their cognitive ability. It is not about how fast they can run or how many push-ups they can do. It is about educating and making accessible the enjoyment of a lifetime activity that improves their quality of life.

If you have any questions, comments, or concerns, do not hesitate to contact me. We need to work together to help our children with disabilities. I want to know what works for your children. I want to know how you did it. Help me be a better educator and leader for our children, and I will do the same for you. Enjoy this special time with your children.

Yours in health,

David

To better understand this book and the Exercise Connection Program, it is important to understand the foundation behind its components. The *Five Components of Physical Fitness for Children with Autism Spectrum Disorders©* (Five Components) was designed by David S. Geslak to meet the needs of our children and better educate the parents and children on physical fitness.

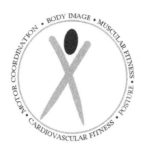

For over 20 years, schools have been educating our youth and parents about the components of fitness: (1) cardiovascular fitness, (2) muscular endurance, (3) muscular strength, (4) flexibility, and (5) body composition. These components were the foundations on which many exercise programs were built. However, over the past 20 years our children's bodies and environments have changed. On a positive note, many new styles of exercise and exercise programs have been introduced recently: for example, yoga, Pilates, and video game exercises. Due to an increase in technology, most of our children are less active with daily tasks, and exercise is no longer a priority.

A child with autism has unique needs that the antiquated components of fitness do not address. It is time that we give children with autism, their parents, and the professionals who work with them, the education needed to make physical activity a priority. As you begin to understand the Five Components, you will see that they meet the needs of all children, irrespective to color, shape, size, or ability. The Five Components will help you as an educator to better educate children with special needs, their parents, and the professionals who work with them. It focuses on the specific needs of the special needs population. Physical exercise is not a priority for either typical or special needs children, but the importance of exercise for the physical and cognitive development of children should not be underestimated.

The Five Components are (1) Body Image, (2) Posture, (3) Motor Coordination, (4) Muscular Fitness, and (5) Cardiovascular Fitness. All of the components from the President's Challenge are embedded within the new Five Components. However, the focus of these new components is on defining and prioritizing what you will be teaching the children and how you will educate the parents and professionals who work with the children.

Body Image

An individual's concept of his/her body and its parts

Within body image there are two focuses: body composition and body awareness. Body composition is defined as the percentage of fat, muscle, and bone in the body. Usually it's expressed as a ratio of lean mass to fatty mass. Lean mass includes muscle, bone, skin, internal organs, and body water. Fatty mass is mostly composed of body fat (subcutaneous fat), as well as internal essential fat that surrounds the organs. Body composition will typically be displayed as either a percentage of fat (body fat percentage or % fat) or as a percentage of lean body mass (LBM).

Body awareness, or proprioception, is the internal sense that recognizes where your body parts are without having to look at them. This is vital to working with every child. If children do not understand where their feet are, or the difference between the left and right hand, it can be difficult to teach them any type of exercise, sport, or activity. While the concept of body awareness may seem very basic, it is overlooked in many fitness programs, especially in programs for children with autism.

Body composition testing is not often done in schools because of the negativity associated with being perceived as overweight or obese. If we continue to ignore body composition, how will we educate children and parents about what is a healthy body weight or body fat percentage?

Within this book you will not learn how to do body composition testing. However, all the exercises in the book will help to improve the body composition of your child, yourself or the children you work with.

Posture

Any position in which the body resides

For posture you are educating and teaching exercises based on balance, static, and dynamic flexibility. Balance is the ability to assume and maintain any body position against the force of gravity. Maintenance of balance results from the interaction of the muscles as they work to keep the body on its base. Also, referring back to Body Image, think of body circumferences, and the physical balance of the body. Are the legs and arms are the same size, etc? Also, can the children perform certain activities with each side of the body (i.e., kick a ball or throw a ball)? Each body part should be relative in size and function.

Flexibility is traditionally demonstrated by sitting down, spreading legs, touching toes, or some form of stretch with limited body movement. Static flexibility is the range of motion of a joint when a body segment is passively moved (e.g., by an exercise partner) and held in position. Flexibility is beneficial to children and can be practiced daily by providing more than a "stretch," but also sensory integration and proprioception. Dynamic flexibility is something we all do every day—moving and stretching. Think of it as reaching up high, on the tips of your toes to get a dish out of a cabinet, or squatting down low to go under the garage door before it closes. Dynamic flexibility is the range of motion that can be achieved by actively moving a body segment using muscle actions. Dynamic flexibility is an important ability underlying many gross motor skills, and is important for developing speed and power.

When people think of posture, they automatically assume an upright position in a chair or a standing position. While these positions help with better musculoskeletal alignment and internal function, they do not define posture.

Our children's bodies move constantly throughout the day, sometimes intentionally and many times unconsciously. No matter the purpose, posture plays a part in helping to improve a child's health.

Static and dynamic flexibility can be taught in both a group class and in a one-on-one training setting. These exercises should be incorporated into each class to help build consistency and routine within the program, to build the child's confidence, and to make the child more successful.

Motor Coordination

The ability of the body to integrate the action of the muscles to accomplish a specific movement, or series of skilled movements, in the most efficient manner

Coordination is defined as a skill and not a component of fitness in the President's Challenge testing protocol. Motor coordination does help to improve the skill of an athlete or anyone involved in sports, but it can also show the strength of the brain. The brain is made "smarter" not only in academics, but also through the movement of the body. Movement is an important component in a child's cognitive development.

Did you know that a child who can skip can read better than a child who cannot? Skipping is critical because it involves both hemispheres of the brain. Your left hemisphere is active when you use the right side of your body, and your right hemisphere is active when you use the left side of your body. The inability to skip is an indicator that both hemispheres are not working in harmony as they should.

There are many activities that can help improve gross motor coordination. These activities should be practiced daily. Fine-motor movement is also important, and is typically practiced in occupational therapy. This book primarily provides you with gross motor movement activities, however, if you want to incorporate fine motor activities into your child's program, do it!

When you think of motor coordination, I want you to think of large gross motor movements, such as skipping, running, and walking. But also think of the motor coordination and planning necessary to carry out those movements—eye-foot coordination and eye-hand coordination.

Eye-hand coordination refers to the ability to use the eyes and hands together to accomplish a task. An example of a task requiring eye-hand coordination is catching a baseball.

Eye-foot coordination refers to the ability to use the eyes and the feet together to accomplish a task. An example of a task requiring eye-foot coordination is kicking a soccer ball.

Motor coordination is an essential part of a child's development, and each day some form of coordination should be incorporated into his/her program. The activities, sports, or tasks you ask the child to do may not look ideal, but remember the child is using the brain as much as other parts of the body to accomplish the task.

Muscular Fitness

The strength and endurance of the muscles

Muscular strength is the maximal amount of force that one can generate in an isolated movement of a single muscle group. Lifting heavy weights once or twice maximally facilitates the measurement of muscular strength. Muscular endurance is the ability of the muscles to apply a submaximal force repeatedly or to sustain a submaximal contraction for a certain period of time. Common muscular endurance exercises are sit-ups, push-ups, chin-ups, or lifting weights 10–15 times in succession.

Muscular strength and muscular endurance have traditionally been kept separate in our education of the human body. This separation causes confusion.

Should you let small children lift heavy weights? No. Could it stunt their growth? Possibly, but more importantly, it can enhance their risk of injury. However, you see this happening every day in schools – children carry backpacks that are too heavy for their body weight or doing "heavy work" to reduce self-stimulatory and maladaptive behaviors. The way our children are physically assessed focuses on quantity (How many push-ups can you do? How fast can you run), not on the quality of movement.

Muscular fitness is a vital part of a child's daily lifestyle and should be taught with correct form and mechanics. Being fit can also help improve sensory integration and proprioception. If you (or any instructor) are unclear about the amount of weight to use in an activity, always choose the least amount. If there is confusion about how to perform a certain exercise or how to use a piece of equipment, then don't do it until the answers are clear.

Combining these vital components of education about the body will help to improve your and your children's understanding of the importance of muscular fitness.

Cardiovascular Fitness

The efficiency of the heart, lungs, and vascular system in delivering oxygen to the working muscles so that prolonged physical work can be maintained

Cardiovascular fitness is often categorized as one of the most important components of a fitness program. The heart is what keeps us moving; it must be strong and powerful.

For children, cardiovascular activity can be one of the most challenging components of an exercise program. When you think of cardio, what do you envision – the treadmill, running, or maybe riding the exercise bike? These are all great examples.

However, for some children getting them to initially stand and walk is an accomplishment. Do not force a child to run if he/she is not ready. If the child is used to sitting on the computer or playing video games, walking will initially provide an improvement in cardiovascular fitness. Your challenge as a parent and instructor will then be up to find motivators that keep the child moving.

If you have access to a pool, remember that along with improving the cardiovascular system, swimming can also help calm a child's sensory system. Even a small amount of movement has cardiovascular benefits, and can turn into a large amount over time.

In order to implement an exercise program, it is important to understand the procedures involved. Staying consistent with procedures and routine will be helpful not only to you as a parent, teacher or instructor, but more importantly to the children with autism.

Here are four elements that should be practiced daily within your child's exercise program:

1. Structure

Children need structure and routine. Many research studies are done on children with autism to understand what can be done to minimize their maladaptive behaviors and allow them to lead a typical lifestyle. Structure is a critical component to success for children with autism and should be generalized across multiple settings (e.g., classroom, gym class, speech therapy, occupational therapy, home).

If you attempt to put children with autism into an unstructured environment, you can expect an unstructured response. Even after establishing structure, however, you may encounter maladaptive behaviors from the children when first implementing an exercise program. Keep moving forward and follow the remaining elements!

Maladaptive behaviors in children with autism are often caused by entering a novel environment. Children with autism may not have participated in the services that you or your organization provides. The structure may be something to which they are not accustomed; however, the value it provides is priceless. If parents are uneducated about the importance of providing a structured environment, this is your opportunity to educate them. Continue to change the lives of these children, because even if they can't tell you, they are thankful for your efforts.

The Exercise Connection Program utilizes 4 stations to teach the exercises and activities. Set up 4 cones throughout your room and each cone, or station, represents a new activity or exercise. Have the children rotate through the stations. The amount of time at the station will vary depending on the amount of time per class/session and repetitions per exercise may vary depending on the number of children.

2. Supports

Some children with autism may not entirely comprehend your verbal instructions. They may understand only a few words in a sentence that you say. For example, if you said, "Johnny, lift your right knee over the hurdle and then your left." The child may have only understood the words "Johnny," or "left," or "Johnny...right...left." You can see how this scenario may become confusing or frustrating for the child.

Visual supports, such as a photo showing a person or character performing the action, will help the child to succeed in the program. The use of visuals will not hinder a child's development and understanding of the activity or skill the child is being asked to perform. If you are working with a new child, supports can make a world of difference in how the child performs tasks and behaviors accurately and sufficiently.

If you are working with a child who does not need visual supports, then it is not necessary to use them. However, you should always have visual supports in place and ready if needed. Think of a "to-do" list. If you show the child your expectations, he/she may be more inclined to finish the activities when they are presented visually and the child can physically cross them off.

Whether you are teaching an exercise to a child or to a senior citizen, it is helpful to have them watch you as you model the activity or exercise. If you can't do/model the exercise yourself, then don't expect your student to do it.

Visual supports include:

- Picture schedules
- Station cards – describing activity or exercise
- Countdown boards
- First/Then boards
- White boards
- Timers (stopwatch, sand timer)

3. Motivation

Whether you are a parent, teacher, or assistant to a child with autism, your positive attitude may be the most important component in any program or therapy. Children can understand whether you are genuine in your actions. They may not be able to completely process what you are saying, but your non-verbal communication tells them more than you realize.

If your role is overseeing the exercise program and the assistance to the children, be sure to focus on your staff. If their non-verbal communication is telling you they need a break or they are frustrated, find a means to give them a break.

We are all positive role models for the children and they need our leadership.

4. Patience

Children with autism do not process things the way a neuro-typical child does. If you expect that they will, you are setting yourself up for failure. However, just because they learn differently it does not contradict my philosophy of "seeing the children for their capabilities, not their disabilities."

If you provide the structure, supports, and motivation, these children can and will do what you ask. Executing an exercise or activity may not happen in a day, a week, or a month, but one day success will come and when it does, it will be amazing!

I worked with a student for nearly five months trying to get him to do a jumping jack (feet only), given on page 31. I tried visuals, verbal prompts, non-verbal prompts, and modeling, everything I could think of. I felt like giving up. Then in the sixth month he did it!

Don't ever give up.

1. Body Part Identification

Goal: To improve the knowledge of body parts and basic neural-motor coordination.

- Body part identification can be done in large groups or individually. In a group setting, it is best not to have the children face each other so they do not imitate the action of the other children.

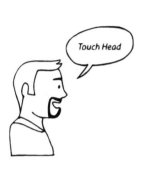
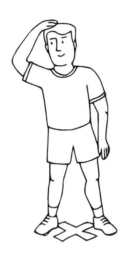

Touch Head

As they improve start to teach them specific muscles or groups of muscles. Ex. "Show me your biceps."

How To

- Give the child verbal instructions. If the child is unable to process the instruction, show the child the visual support card.
- If they begin to understand then help them to distinguish between the right and left sides of the body. e.g., right hand.

How Many

- This should be practiced everyday if the child cannot understand body parts.
- Practice for up to 5 minutes.

Coaching Tips

- Do not rush your child, give them time to process your request.
- When asking the child to touch the appropriate body part, it is important that you <u>do not</u> model the action. It is important to find out if the child can verbally or visually understand what you are asking.
- Show excitement at the correct response!

2. The Pretzel

Goal: To engage both hemishpheres of the brain and while doing it trying to calm and refocus the child.

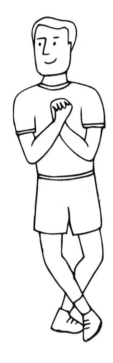

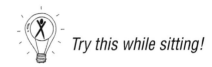

Try this while sitting!

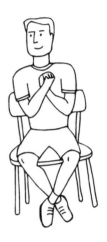

How To

- Have the child begin by crossing one foot over the other. Next, have the child extend his arms out and have the backs of the hands touching with thumbs down. Then bring the right or left arm over and interlock the fingers. Finally, have them bring their hands toward their body so they rest on their chest. While doing it have them place their tongue on the roof of their mouth.

How Many

- Have the child hold the position for up to 60 seconds. When beginning they may only be able to hold for 10 seconds.
- You may have to help interlock the fingers.
- If they don't put their tongue on the roof of the mouth, at first, it is ok.

3. Crossover March

Goal: To consecutively cross the midline of the body using opposite arm(s) and leg(s) while improving motor coordination.

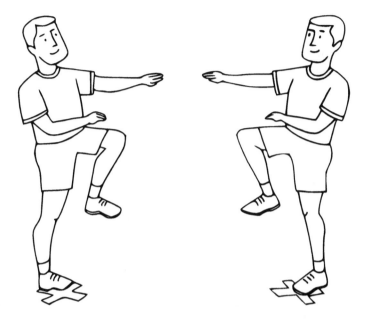

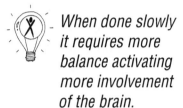

When done slowly it requires more balance activating more involvement of the brain.

How To

- This exercise can help improve walking and running mechanics. Make an "X" on the ground or use a cone as a visual marker for the child to stand. It is best to model this exercise, once, for the child.

- The goal is for the child to march in place, bringing his/her right knee up and touching it with his/her left hand, and then bringing the left knee up and touching it with his/her right hand.

How Many

- Shoot for 6 consecutive touches and then go for more. Have the child count while they do it too!

Coaching Tips

- You may need to physically prompt them to touch the appropriate hand to knee. Before a full prompt try tapping the appropriate leg and knee.

- If they can't perform it in place, have them try walking in a circle or forwards and backwards. I have had a lot of success with this approach.

4. Log Exercises

Goal: To help improve the individual's proprioception while improving the flexibility and range of motion of the posterior shoulder girdle.

How To

- It is important that you model how to get onto the log. When the child squats down to sit on the log you may have to adjust the log during the process. It is important that the butt is on the far end of the log and that the child then lays back. The back of the head should be on the log and in a neutral position or the neck relaxed.

How Many

- Begin with 30 seconds for the general stretch. If they want to stay on longer it is fine; they are in a safe position.
- When performing the arm actions, have them perform 8-12 repetitions.

General Stretch

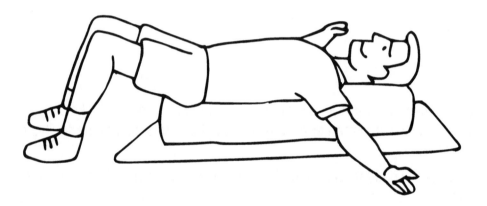

 These exercises are like self massages and can help reduce tension in the neck. Give it a try mom and dad!

Coaching Tips

- Have palms facing up
- If the hands are not on the ground that is ok. Don't force them down; this means that the muscles of the neck and shoulder girdle are tight. This will happen naturally; keep practicing and watch to see the improvement.

Claps

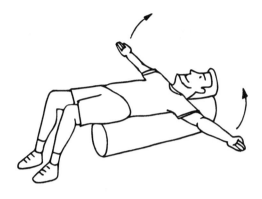

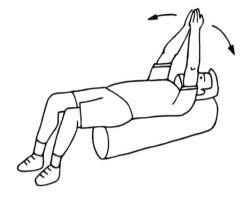

Start   **Finish**

Angels in the Snow

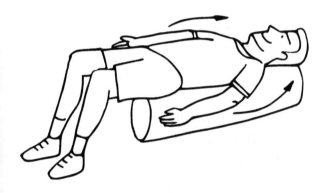

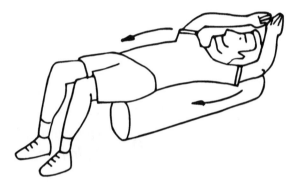

Start   **Finish**

Coaching Tips

- To maintain stability, make sure the knees are bent with the feet flat on the ground.
- The arm movements may take some time for the child to perform; try moving one arm at a time before using both arms.
- These exercises can be done everyday before and after workout.

5. Calf Stretch

Goal: To improve flexibility and relax the muscles of the calves.

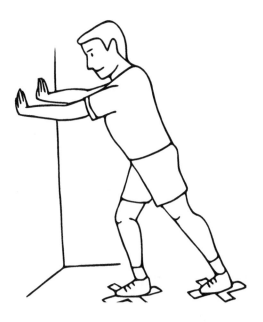

 Research has shown that stretching the calf muscles has a link to verbal skills and help with communication in speech impaired children and children with autism.

How To

- Have the child step forward with the left leg keeping the right leg about 12-18 inches behind (length depends on size of child). Toes should point forward while hands can be placed on hips, wall, chair or a stable object. Next, slowly bend the left leg forward while keeping the back heel flat. Repeat on opposite leg.

How Many

- Hold for up to 30 seconds on each leg.
- If the child bounces into the stretch, have him do up to 20 bounces.

Coaching Tips

- Keep toes pointing forward.
- Back heel always flat.
- Have the child count while holding the position.

6. Hip Extensions

Goal: To improve the function and development of the gluteal and hamstring muscles.

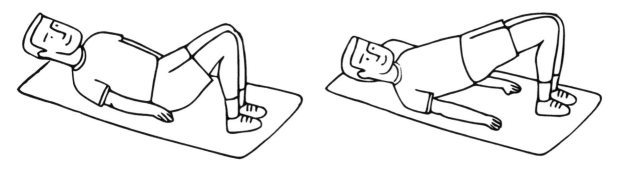

Start   **Finish**

 Hip extensions will help to reduce the risk of low back pain by developing the gluteal (butt) and hamstring muscles.

How To

- Have the children lie on their back with knees bent, feet flat and neck relaxed. Then have the children lift their butt up so the knee, hip and shoulder are in a straight line. Control the movement on the way down and repeat.

How Many

- Perform 2-4 sets for 6-15 repetitions each.

Coaching Tips

- Try not to let the butt hit the ground, helping to reduce the risk of injury, while challenging the muscles.
- If the child begins doing this exercise fast, that's ok, they're moving! Each time work to make it a more controlled movement.

7. Mini-Band Exercises

Goal: To improve the strength and endurance of the adductors and abductors (muscles of the hips and inner thighs) while improving proprioception and body awareness.

Lateral (Side) Steps

Forward Skater Walks

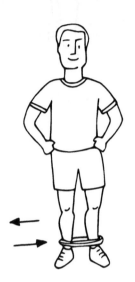

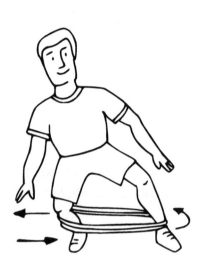

 Always use a lighter, or less tense, mini-band. The goal is not to make the exercise too hard, because it will restrict the range of motion, not making the movements as natural as possible.

How To

- Have the child put the mini-band around both feet and bring it just above the ankles. If wearing shorts it may be helpful to put the band over the socks.
- Next have the child take a step to the right, with the right foot, and have the left foot go to where the right foot was. Repeat for a few steps and then move in the opposite direction.

How Many

- Perform each movement to the right and left side or leading with the right and left leg; 1-4 sets with 6-12 repetitions on each side

Coaching Tips

- Always keep tension on the band and do not drag the feet on the ground.
- Have the toes point forward with the knees slightly bent.

8. Single Leg Balance

Goal: To improve balance, laterality, and strength of each leg.

How To

- The single leg balance should be practiced on both sides. The child should be asked verbally, or shown by use of a visual support card, to support his/her weight on the appropriate foot.

How Many

- Goal is for the child to hold the position for 3 seconds on each leg.
- Perform 1-5 sets for 3-15 seconds on each leg.

Coaching Tips

- Try to have a slight knee bend.
- Arms out can help.
- Eyes focusing on an object may also help.

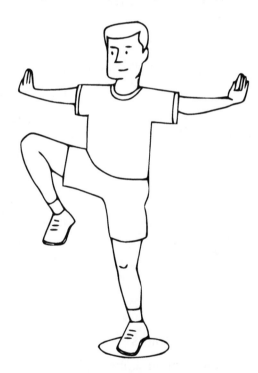

 If your child can do this have him try brushing his teeth on one leg.

9. Ladder Drills

Goal: To improve foot-eye coordination and visual motor association. Three exercises can be practiced: 2-In Forward, 2-In Lateral, 2-Foot Hops.

How To

- To help the child perform this exercise, modeling should be used. You can place footprints on the ground, as shown in the example. Also show the child a visual support card that describes the exercise.

- When demonstrating, walk through the exercise, using big body movements to show the child what you want the child to do. You want the child to place each foot into the four squares with the same pattern of movement (i.e., right foot, then left foot).

- You are asking the child to perform this exercise two different ways, leading with the right foot (as in the photo) and then leading with the left foot.

How Many

- Successfully perform 1 set of 4 squares of each pattern.

2-IN FORWARD...

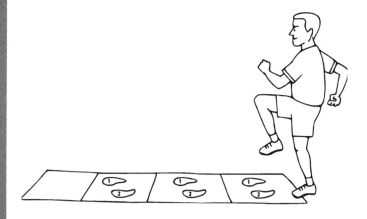

 Ladders can be made with masking tape to use indoors or sidewalk chalk outdoors.

Coaching Tips

- Instead of using footprints you can also use colors.
- If it doesn't look perfect, that's ok! Keep encouraging and practicing. Getting them moving is half the battle.

How To

- To help the child complete this exercise, modeling should be used. Place footprints on the ground, as shown in the example. Also show the child a visual support card that describes the exercise.

- When demonstrating walk through the exercise, using big body movements, to show the child what you want them to do. You want the child to place each foot into the four squares with the same pattern of movement (i.e., right foot, then left foot). The feet should not cross!

- The child should be moving laterally (side-to-side). Have the child face you or use an object to help them put their feet into the correct position.

- You are asking the child to perform this exercise two different ways, leading with the left foot (as in the above photo) and then leading with the right foot.

- The child must complete all four squares for proper evaluation.

2-IN LATERAL...

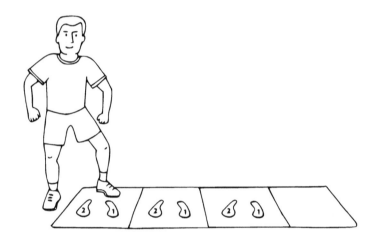

 Moving laterally not only challenges the muscles of the ankles, knees and hips but also the brain.

Coaching Tips

- Holding their hands, facing you, may help them to understand that you want them to move side-to-side.

- Tell the children to make up their own pattern, this will encourage them to take ownership of the exercise.

- To help the child complete this exercise, modeling should be used. You can place footprints on the ground, as shown in the example. Also show the child a visual support card that describes the exercise.

- When demonstrating, jump through the exercise slowly, showing the child what you want them to do. You want the child to jump with feet together into the four squares. Speed is not important. Getting through the pattern is what matters.

- You are asking the child to perform this exercise two different ways, hopping forward and hopping backward. If the child looks backward when hopping in that direction, that is fine.

2-FOOT HOPS...

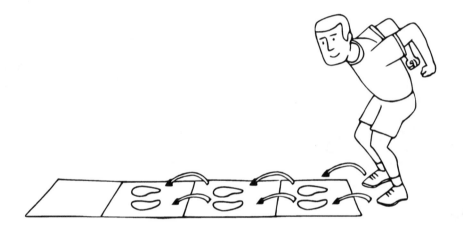

Coaching Tips

- As you ask them to jump forward, face them with feet in the ladder, and jump backwards.
- Be patient; the ability to jump is very challenging for our children.
- You can try putting a small box or book for them to jump to and down from.

10. Dot Drills

Goal: To improve gross motor coordination and for strengthening the muscles of the ankles, knees and hips while improving the knowledge of letters.

Double Leg Jumps   **Single Leg Jumps**

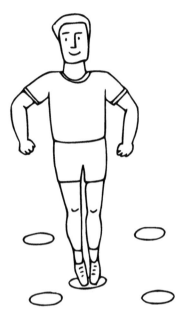
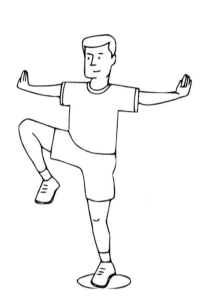

 Practice spelling these letters:

N, M, W, X, Z, C, D.

How To

- Make 5 dots on the ground using masking tape, chalk or spray paint. Arrange the dots between 1-2 feet apart similar to the photos above.

- Always have the child start with double leg jumps. Have them starting on the appropriate dot to the letter they are going to "spell." For example, if spelling "M," the child would begin on the bottom left dot. If spelling "X" one foot would be on bottom left, the other on bottom right. Then jump to the middle with both feet and finish the way they started at the top two dots.

How Many

- Correctly spell each letter once. Once able, you can repeat for up to 5 sets per session.

Coaching Tips

- If the child doesn't jump and walks to spell the letter that is great! Their brain is processing the letters in another way. The jumping may take time…

- If it becomes easy for the child have them try jumping the letters on one leg.

11. Hurdles Drills (Over and Under)

Goal: To improve lower body flexibility while improving proprioception and body awareness.

How To

Over

- Set the hurdle(s) height in such a way that they do not go above the knee cap.
- Have the child step over leading with the right or left foot, focusing on lifting the knee up. The back leg should follow and the knee should lift up, the leg should not drape over.

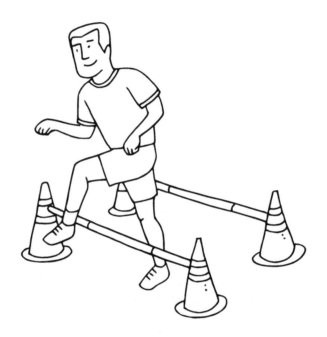

 Try the exercises with the arms overhead; you will automatically engage the abdominal muscles making it challenge the body and brain.

How Many

- The child should complete one series of 2-4 hurdles consecutively without hitting hurdle or knocking any over.
- Add more sets when the child is ready.

Under

- When beginning it is appropriate to set the hurdle(s) at the tallest height. As flexibility and proprioception improves you can begin to lower the height.
- Have the child begin standing with the right or left shoulder facing the front the hurdle.
- Next, have the child put their right or left leg under the hurdle on the opposite side of which they stand.
- Then have the child get their butt down, chest and eyes up and go under the hurdle.
- Make sure to repeat with the opposite leg.

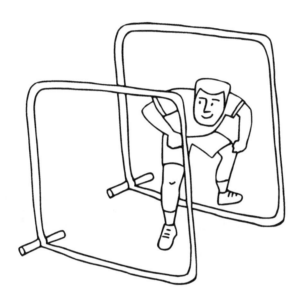

How Many

- A child should complete one series of 2-4 hurdles consecutively without hitting hurdle or knocking any over.
- Add more sets when the child is ready.

Coaching Tips

- If you do an exercise leading with the right foot or from the right side of the body, always practice it on the opposite side.
- When going under you may have to physically maneuver the hurdle so they don't hit it. Remember, it's about encouraging the activity, not setting the child up for failure.
- If they go slow over the hurdle that's even better. Doing this improves single leg balance.

12. Jumping Jack (Feet Only)

Goal: To improve motor coordination and sensory integration.

How To

- The child will not actually be crossing midline; however, the goal is for the child's feet to meet at midline.
- To help the child complete this assessment, modeling should be used, as well as "Xs" or markers placed on the ground.

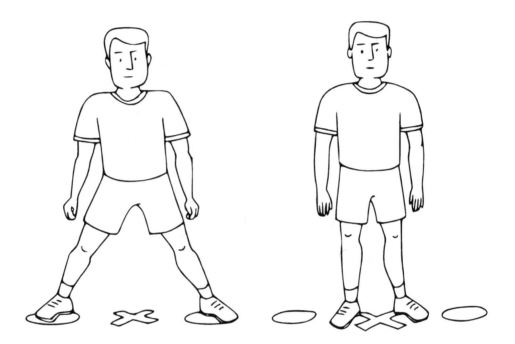

How Many

- Perform 1-5 sets of 1-25 repetitions.

Coaching Tips

- Use a favorite picture or character for them to jump on.
- You can try this using the exercise ladder.
- If it helps to use the arms while jumping then have the child do it. Sometimes processing two movements at once can be too challenging, but it is important to remember that every child is unique and learns differently.

13. Ball Catch (Large & Small)

Goal: To improve eye-hand coordination and ocular pursuit.

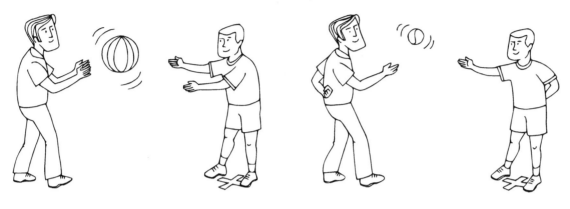

 An overhand toss can be very threatening for the child. Always begin with an underhand toss, starting close together.

How To

- The child should stand facing you approximately 4–6 feet away. Marking an "X" on the ground with masking tape, or using a cone, may help to put the child in position. You should then throw a ball (soccer, basketball, or a ball similar in size) to the child using an underhand toss. The child should attempt to catch the ball using fingers and hands only.

- When using a small ball (baseball or another ball similar in size) the set-up procedure is the same as the set-up procedure for the large ball. However, you can give the child a physical prompt by touching the appropriate hand to catch with, or you can model or physically prompt the child to put the opposite hand behind his/her back. The child should attempt to catch the ball using his/her hand and fingers. Three trials are given.

Coaching Tips

- Use a ball that is comfortable for the child; a ball that is squishy or visually stimulating is very good.

- Practicing throwing and catching with the non-dominant hand can help to improve the dominant hand.

14. Wall Push-Up

Goal: To improve upper body muscular fitness.

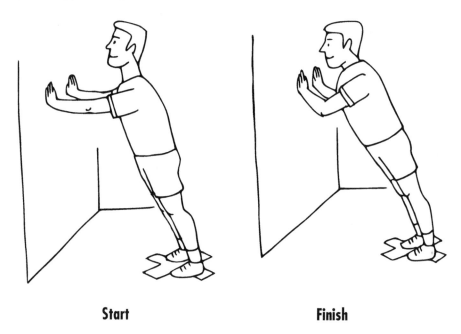

| Start | Finish |

How To

- Place a visual marker, "X" or line 2-3 feet from the wall depending on the size of the child.
- Next have the child place their hands on the wall. You may also need to place a tape or a marker on the wall of where their hands should be placed.
- Then have the child lean their chest or body towards the wall, with the elbows close to the body not wide, and then push themselves up.
- Modeling this exercise will be very important.

How Many

- 1-4 sets of 3-20 repetitions.
- When beginning set an achievable amount for the child.

Coaching Tips

- Encourage keeping the elbows closer to the body than wide and away from the body.
- If the child goes too fast or too slow, encourage a proper cadence by counting or using music with a beat.

15. Wall Push Up with Clap

Goal: To improve upperbody muscular fitness and coordination.

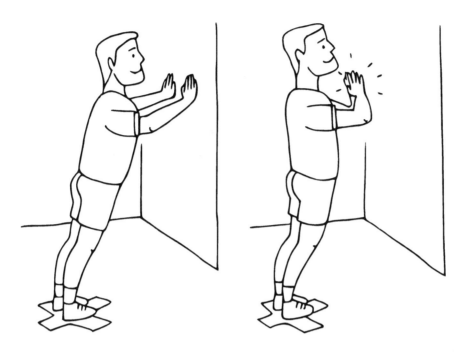

How To

- Place a visual marker, "X" or line 2-3 feet from the wall depending on size of the child.
- Next have the child place their hands on the wall. You may also need to place a tape or a marker on the wall of where their hands should be placed.
- Then have the child lean their chest or body towards the wall, elbows close to the body not wide, and then push themselves up.
- As they push up, the child should remove his hands from the wall and clap. Then start again.
- Modeling this exercise will be very important.

How Many

- 1-4 sets of 3-20 repetitions.
- When beginning set an achievable amount for the child.

Coaching Tips

- For some children this may be easier to teach because of the clapping.

16. Push-Up Hold

Goal: To improve the strength and endurance of the abdominals, arm, glutes/hamstrings, and shoulder girdle.

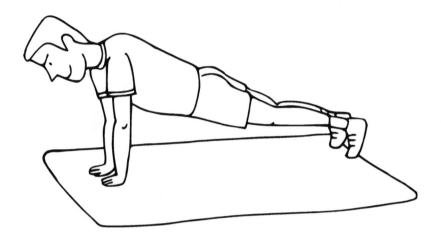

How To

- Have the child start on the ground on their hands and knees.
- Next, make sure the hands are flat on ground or mat with the chest directly over the hands.
- Then, have them put one leg straight back, with the toes or ball of foot on ground; then follow with the other leg.
- Be patient, this is a challenging exercise for the entire body.

How Many

- 1-3 sets for 5-20 seconds.

Coaching Tips

- You want to picture a straight line through the shoulder, hip, knee and ankle.
- In the beginning you may have to physically prompt their hips up to prevent them from sinking.
- Start slowly, holding between 3 – 8 seconds, and gradually increasing the length of time.

17. Elbows 'n' Toes

Goal: To strengthen the muscles of the abdominal, glutes, hamstrings and shoulder girdle.

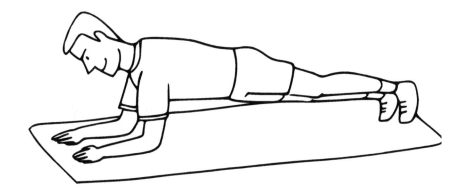

 This exercise works the entire body and can be more effective and safer than a traditional sit-up or crunch.

How To

- To help the child complete this assessment, modeling should be used. If needed, show the child a visual support card that describes the exercise.
- Have the child begin with forearms and palms flat against the floor. Next, have the child place the legs straight back, toes pushing into the floor. You want the child to maintain a flat back (the butt is not too high or sinking).

How Many

- 1-4 set for 5-20 seconds.

Coaching Tips

- Have the child try holding a push-up position first.
- If the child can perform the exercise, try tapping them on their shoulders, sides of the torso and legs as they do it. This further challenges the muscles of the abdominals.
- Make sure their neck stays relaxed, eyes looking at the ground.

18. Medicine Ball Series

Goal: To improve the muscular fitness of the muscles of the chest, shoulders and arms.

Medicine Ball Chop

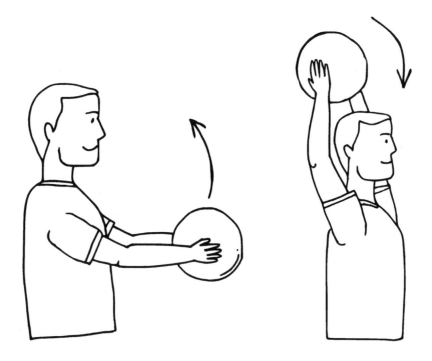

How To

- Begin with the ball away from chest and with the arm straight. Slowly lift ball overhead keeping arms straight.
- When bringing the ball down, slowly lower keeping arms straight.

How Many

- Perform 1-3 sets of 3 – 12 repetitions.

Coaching Tips

- Always begin with a lighter weight medicine ball.
- You may have to guide their arms into the correct position for the first few repetitions.

MB Overhead Press

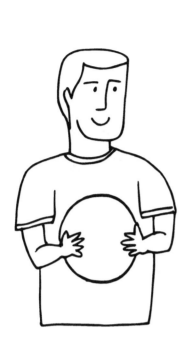 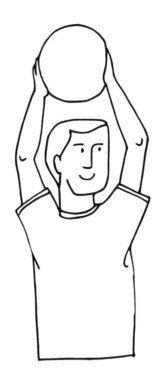

How To

- Begin with the ball at chest level, both hands firmly on the sides of the ball.
- Push or press the ball over the head with the arm near full extension.

Coaching Tips

- To help the child reach full extension have them hit your hand or an object with the ball above the head.
- The knees should have a slight bend and their upper body should be standing tall, not hunched over in any way.

MB Partner Chest Press

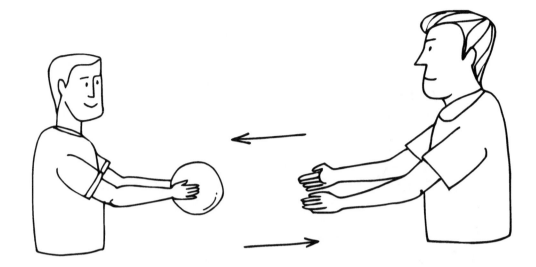

 An advanced exercise is medicine ball chest passes, similar to chest passes with a basketball.

How To

- Have the child begin with the ball at chest level, hand firmly gripping the sides of the ball.
- Partner should be standing in front of them, with arm about 2 feet from the ball at chest level.
- Have the child touch your hands or an object and return ball to starting position. Ball should be kept at chest level through the entire movement.

Coaching Tips

- If the ball starts dropping through the movement, replace with a lighter weight ball.
- Counting backwards (ex, 3..2..1) can better help the child understand when they are finished.

19. Funky Running

(Wide Run/Tight Rope, Least Amount/Many Steps,
Quiet Feet/Loud Feet, Fast Arms/No Arms)

Goal: To improve gross motor coordination that will help the mechanics of running, walking and large gross motor activities.

*This is a series of running forms that ideally should be practiced together. Try doing them in pairs (i.e. first Wide Run then Tight Rope, etc.). If they cannot be practiced all at once, it is fine. Choose the ones that the child may like and then gradually try the others.

How To

- Pick a distance that is realistic for your child to run/walk and use cones, two objects or lines on the ground that give a start and end point.
- If you have a start and stop visual support card, place it at the appropriate location.
- To have the child begin the exercise it is important to use the same count down and cadence. For example, "Ready…set..go," "Down….set….hike," or "3..2..1..go!"
- If auditory processing is tough for the child, try using an arm movement to start the exercise. For example, Arm begins up the arm and the child starts when it begins to come down. Be sure to demonstrate this for the child.
- Modeling each of these exercises is important.

How Many

- 1-10 set(s) of 5-20 yards of each run.

Wide Run

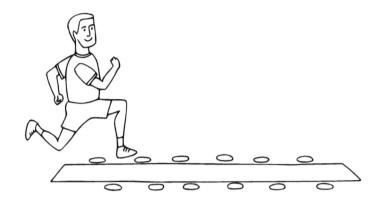

Coaching Tips

- If it looks funny…that's a good thing.
- Encourage getting the "knees up" as they run.

Tight Rope Run

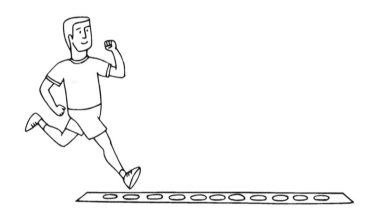

Coaching Tips

- Footprints on the ground will help (as pictured) as well as a line on the ground.
- A more advanced exercise you could try is doing this on a curb. Use caution; start with walking, jogging and then running.

Least Amount of Steps

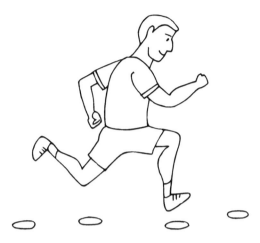

Coaching Tips

- It should almost look like they are leaping or reaching to step on something.
- Place visual markers a distance between 3-5 feet apart to reach to, depending on the child's size and ability.

Many Steps as Possible

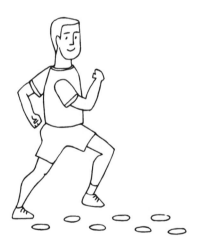

Coaching Tips

- Emphasize getting the "knees up" as they run; sometimes the child may shuffle feet across the ground.
- Watch what the arms do. Are they moving in opposition? Are they just hanging by the sides? When the child is ready then start to talk about arm action.

Loud Feet

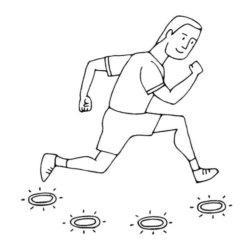

- You don't want them stomping their way to the finish. Make sure they are trying to run.
- If they are jumping to do it, that's ok.

Quiet Feet

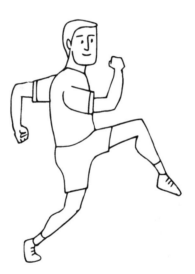

- Tell child to "Be quiet like a cat."
- Have them start by standing on their tip-toes.

Fast Arms

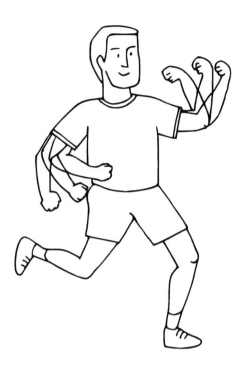

 If the child is having trouble, take the legs out of it. Have him sit on the ground, legs stretched forward, and move the arms fast. When ready move back to the feet.

Coaching Tips

- Use the phrase "chin-hip" as they run. You want the hands to move in opposition from the chin down to the hip. You do not want the hands moving across the body.

- Even if they walk, that is ok; the focus here is on arm action.

No Arms

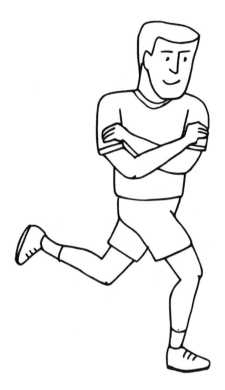

 When running forward if their torso/ upper body moves side to side a lot, this can signify weak abdominals and midsection.

Coaching Tips

- Remember, make all these exercises playful and fun.
- As they continue to improve then start coaching with lifting their knees.

20. Treadmill

Goal: To improve cardiovascular fitness.

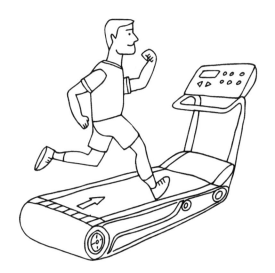

 Don't be afraid to put on their favorite TV show to watch or music while they do the treadmill. We do it at the gym, why shouldn't they?

How To

- Begin by having the child stand on the treadmill and then starting the treadmill around 1 mph. The child may be scared of it.
- Gradually increase the speed as they become more accustomed to it. Faster is not always better, in terms of improving losing weight either.
- Make sure the child holds on the handle bars if they feel uncomfortable. Also, be sure to clip the emergency turn off clip to their shirt or pants.
- If there are many buttons on the machine the child may want to explore or press them all. Cover up the ones that could cause problems, like the "Stop" button.

How Many

- 5 – 30 minutes.
- Begin with walking and slowly increase the speed to a run.

Coaching Tips

- If they are having trouble staying on the treadmill, stand behind the child with your legs on the sides of the treadmill, to prevent them from trying to step off.
- Be the leader, have them watch you do it for 5 minutes and then have them try. "FIRST mom....THEN Johnny."
- Sometimes watching the tread move is more exciting than being on it; encourage them to watch it while walking or running on it.
- If the child cannot run, gradually increase the incline of treadmill; this will help to increase caloric burn and improve cardiovascular fitness.

21. Exercise Bike

Goal: To improve cardiovascular fitness while improving motor coordination.

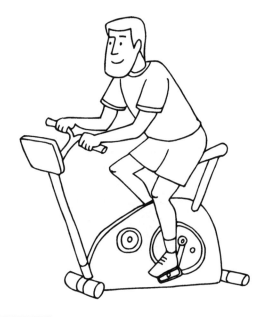

 Children will burn less calories per workout when using a bike compared to a treadmill; however, a bike is safer to use.

How To

- Much like all the exercises, demonstrate what you want the child to do.
- Adjust the seat so that when their knee is not fully extended when turning, there should be a slight knee bend!

How Many

- 5 – 30 minutes.

Coaching Tips

- If they are having trouble pressing down or not wanting to do it, try increasing the resistance; this may give them more sensory feedback.

22. Trampoline

Goal: Improve cardiovascular fitness, while meeting the needs of sensory integration and building the muscular fitness of the muscles of the ankle, knee and hip.

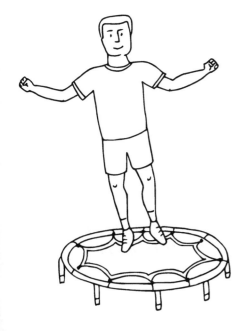

 Have the child try to move their feet, like a jumping jack pattern or shuffling back and forth. Doing so will improve the strength of the ankles, knees and hips while challenging the brain!

How To

- Have the child stand on the trampoline getting on one foot at a time.
- When the child is comfortable ask him/her to "jump" or show a visual support card.

How Many

- Perform 1-5 sets of 10-25 jumps.

Coaching Tips

- If the child is not accustomed to this, holding their hands while jumping may help.

23. Hill Running

Goal: To improve cardiovascular fitness while improving the strength and endurance of the leg muscles and proprioception.

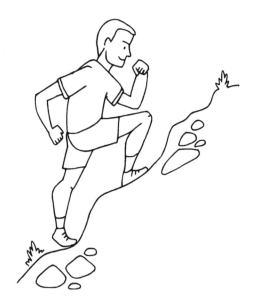

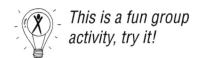
This is a fun group activity, try it!

How To

- Have the child stand at the bottom of a hill on a visual marker. Place a cone or visual marker at the top of the hill or in the middle of the hill to identify a stopping point.
- Use a countdown "3...2...1...GO!" or cadence that the child is familiar with to start.
- If the child walks that is fine, running may take some time, while the walk up a hill is beneficial.
- ALWAYS have the child walk down the hill. Running down the hill can increase risk of injury while putting stress on the knees.

Coaching Tips

- If the child is familiar with the game "tag", have them try to tag up the hill.
- Depending on the size of the hill you may have to set goals before they reach the top. A hill can be very intimidating.

24. Cone Running

Goal: To improve cardiovascular fitness while working on motor planning and following directions.

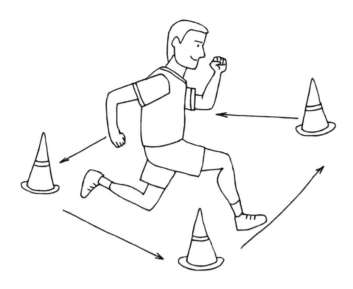

 This same concept can be used to help the children learn to run the bases in baseball. Set up 4 cones in a diamond shape and try it!

How To

- Set up 4 cones at a distance that can be accomplished by the child. You can set up more or less cones if needed.
- Use a cadence familiar to the child to start the activity. Ex. "Ready...Set....Go!
- If the child is walking that is fine, do not push them to run. Let them figure out the pattern, that is half the challenge.

Coaching Tips

- Arrows on the ground can help to show the child which direction you want them to run. Use sidewalk chalk, masking tape of spray paint.
- Run with the child! Don't just talk the talk....walk the walk!

BALANCE

The ability to assume and maintain any body position against the force of gravity. Maintenance of balance results from the interaction of the muscles working to keep the body on its base.

BLOOD PRESSURE

The force of blood against the wall of the arteries and veins, created by the heart as it pumps blood to every part of the body.

BODY IMAGE

The individual's concept of his body and its parts. The concept involves the knowledge of: (a) the physical structure of the body and its parts, (b) the movements and functions of the body and its parts, and (c) the position of the body and its parts in relation to each other and to other subjects.

CARDIOVASCULAR FITNESS

The efficiency of the heart, lungs, and vascular system in delivering oxygen to the working muscles so that prolonged physical work can be maintained.

COORDINATION

The ability of the body to integrate the action of the muscles of the body to accomplish a specific movement or a series of skilled movements in the most efficient manner.

DIRECTIONALITY

An awareness of space outside the body and involves these three elements: (a) knowledge of directions in relation to right and left, in and out, and up and down; (b) the projection of one's self in space; and (c) the judging of distances between objects.

ENDURANCE

The capacity to continue a physical performance over a period of time.

EYE-FOOT COORDINATION

Refers to one's ability to use eyes and feet together to accomplish a task.

EYE-HAND COORDINATION

Refers to one's ability to use eyes and hands together to accomplish a task.

EXERCISE

Physical exertion of sufficient intensity, duration and frequency to achieve or maintain fitness or other health or athletic objectives.

FINE MOTOR COORDINATION

Use of small muscles, resulting from the development of the muscles to the degree that they can perform specific small movements (such as cutting, writing, grasping, etc.

FLEXIBILITY

The range of motion around a joint.

GROSS MOTOR COORDINATION

Results from the development of the skeletal or large muscles to produce efficient total body movement.

HYPERTENSION

Simply a condition in which the blood pressure is chronically elevated above optimal levels. Hypertension is diagnosed in adults when diastolic measurements (blood pressure when the heart is resting) on at least two separate visits average 90 mm Hg or higher, and/or systolic measurements (while the heart is beating) are 140 mm Hg or higher.

KINESTHESIS

One's awareness of muscular movement and expenditure of energy as a skill is performed.

LATERALITY

Internalizing the awareness of the difference between left and right. It is the ability to control the two sides of the body together or separately and is the motor basis for spatial concepts.

MUSCULAR ENDURANCE

The ability of the muscles to apply a submaximal force repeatedly or to sustain a submaximal contraction for a certain period of time.

MUSCULAR FITNESS

The strength and the endurance of the muscles.

MUSCULAR STRENGTH

The maximal amount of force that one can generate in an isolated movement of a single muscle group.

OBESITY

Excessive accumulation of body fat. Obesity may have an adverse effect on health, leading to increased risk of heart disease, type 2 diabetes, certain types of cancer and reduced life expectancy.

OCULAR PURSUIT

The ability of the eyes to work together in following (tracking) a moving object or in focusing from one object to another.

PERCEPTUAL MOTOR SKILLS

Our sensory motor skills are those which indicate the interrelationships between the perceptual or sensory processes and motor activity and the ability of the individual to receive, interpret, and respond accurately to stimuli, either internal or external. Perceptual-motor learning involves all senses: seeing, hearing, touching, tasting, smelling, and moving or kinesthesis.

POSTURE

Any position in which the body resides.

SENSORY INTEGRATION

The normal neurological process of taking in information from one's body and environment through the senses, of organizing and unifying this information, and of using it to plan and execute adaptive responses to different challenges in order to learn and function smoothly in daily life.

SPATIAL ORIENTATION

Involves the ability to select a reference point to stabilize functions and to organize objects into the correct perspective. It involves knowledge of the body and its position, as well as the positions of other people and objects in relation to one's body in space.

VISUAL MOTOR ASSOCIATION

Refers to the ability to successfully integrate visual and motor responses into a physical action. It enables an individual to control movement, and move easily and smoothly from place to place.

References

Capon, Jack. *Book 1: Basic Movement Activities.* CA: Front Row, 1994.

Hannaford, Carla. *Smart Moves: Why Learning is Not All in Your Head.* NC: Great Oceans, 1995.

Kendall, Florence, Elizabeth McCreary, and Patricia Provance. *Muscles: Testing and Function.* 4th ed. Philadelphia: 1993.

Lochbaum, Mark R., Debra J. Crews. 1995. Exercise Prescription for Autistic Populations. 25. no 3:335-336.

Nieman, David C. *Exercise Testing and Prescription: A Health-Related Approach.* 4th ed. CA: Mayfield, 1999.

Rosenthal-Malek, Andrea, and Stella Mitchell. 1997. Brief Report: The Effects of Exercise on the Self-Stimulatory Behaviors and Positive Responding of Adolescents with Autism. *Journal of Autism and Developmental Disorders* 27, no. 2:193-202.

Stock Kranowitz, Carol. The Out-of-Sync Child: Recognizing and coping with sensory integrations dysfunction. New York: Skylight, 1998.

U.S. Department of Health and Human Services. The President's Challenge: Physical Activity & Fitness Awards Program 2004–2005. Indiana: 2004.

David S. Geslak is an autism fitness specialist and has been developing exercise programs for youth and adults with autism spectrum disorders since 2004. He is founder of the Exercise Connection an internationally recognized autism fitness program, adopted in Cairo, Egypt and within autism organizations across the United States.

David began his fitness career as an assistant strength and conditioning coach for the University of Iowa Football Program. Here he learned the importance of individual physical assessments of which he implements on all children no matter, age, size or ability.

When he left Iowa Football he moved back home to Chicago and co-founded Right Fit, a fitness facility with a mission to serving children. Here he began working with children on the autism spectrum. Students of all ages from a school for children with autism, Giant Steps, were coming to Right Fit for their physical education. David wanted to learn more about autism and what the children experienced daily and he left the business to go work as a paraprofessional.

This experience brought him closer to the children and all the teachers and therapists that work with them. Giant Steps then asked David to start their first Special Recreation Program. In 2009 David implemented the program and within 8 months it was featured on ABC 7 news and was able to receive a grant.

Also in 2009 David founded the Exercise Connection with a mission to empower families, educators and physicians to become leaders in health and fitness for their children or the children they work with. He developed an exercise DVD to educate these groups which has been purchased all over the world. He has presented the Exercise Connection Philosophy throughout the United States and internationally.

David is the co-host of *Outspoken with Karon Gibson*, a TV show featured in the Chicagoland area promoting health and wellness for all. He has also been a featured author for the Autism File Magazine and numerous online publications.

David graduated from the University of Iowa with a Bachelors Degree in Health Promotion. He is also a Certified Health Fitness Specialist with the American College of Sports Medicine and a Certified Strength and Conditioning Specialist with the National Strength and Conditioning Association.

Lightning Source UK Ltd.
Milton Keynes UK
UKHW050210070422
401203UK00001B/26